It's Okay

It's Okay:

Living and Loving Through Cancer

Toni Roberts

Editor:
Ellen Gay Leathers-Morrill

Co-Editor:
Terry Ethington

iUniverse, Inc.
New York   Bloomington

It's Okay
Living and Loving Through Cancer

iUniverse books may be ordered through booksellers or by contacting:

*iUniverse
1663 Liberty Drive
Bloomington, IN 47403
www.iuniverse.com
1-800-Authors (1-800-288-4677)*

*ISBN: 978-1-4401-1938-5 (pbk)
ISBN: 978-1-4401-1939-2 (ebk)*

*Author photograph taken by Tom Osborne, The Studio Photography,
Mt. Sterling, KY*

Printed in the United States of America

iUniverse rev. date: 1/19/2009

Dedication

This book is dedicated to Bill, my loving husband whose unconditional love and gentle strength sustained both of us through this trial. For the many painful and sleepless nights that he walked with me, carried me and cradled me, I give him my thanks. Bill's abiding love and companionship has highlighted and punctuated my life with delight, adventure, energy, gentleness, curiosity, strength, and supreme courage. It's been an indescribable joy to be married to someone with whom I have no regrets, no second guesses. There is no place I'd rather be than in his strong, loving arms.

"…I found the one my heart loves. I held him and would not let him go…"   Song of Solomon 3:4

Foreword

When your days are numbered by cancer, people ask why you would spend time writing a book instead of playing with your grandchildren or relishing family moments. It's because this is the book I needed. During my darkest times, I tried to fill my mind with spiritual books that were uplifting and encouraging but discovered that those books were difficult to find. Some of the books about people with cancer made me cry, but mostly they made me feel as if I were going through the disease all over again. I didn't need to go through anyone else's nightmare – I was in the middle of my own. Reading about their experience with cancer put me right back there, receiving chemo, losing hair and being filled with anger and fear. The books didn't teach me how to cope with the cards I'd been dealt. I needed information -- not more misery. I'll show you my darkness just so I can show you how to get out of your own.

I hope this book offers insight on how to live with cancer in a way that makes patients know they'll be okay with their situation. There's a difference in living life waiting to die and living life abundantly.

This book is not just a story about what happened to me. Cancer doesn't just happen to one person. It happens to families, loved ones, friends and communities. More than the details of what happened during that dark time in my life, this story shares what I learned from what happened to us all.

Contents

Chapter 1

Changing Direction

"Consider it pure joy, my brothers, whenever you face trials of many kinds, because you know that the testing of your faith develops perseverance. Perseverance must finish its work so that you may be mature and complete, not lacking anything." James 1:2-4

"That pain I've been having is getting worse, Honey," I yelled into the adjoining room where my husband, Bill, sat in his "man's" den. Our computer stations were near enough to yell across the room at each other yet far enough away to give each of us our alone time. "Now it's going from my abdomen through to my back and making me nauseated. I think it's time I check into getting these gallstones out."

"Okay, Toni. First thing in the morning get an ultrasound with Mike," he yelled back. And that was that. Bill is a doctor and knows how to handle everything. On Tuesday, our good friend and business partner, Mike, would be in his office with his ultrasound equipment. What luck.

Bill is the love of my life, and he's the smartest man I know. He is compassionate and passionate about family evidenced by our three daughters' respect and love for him. Bill is tall, handsome with a chiseled jaw, quick smile, and analytical mind; he is energetic and curious about so many things. Every year of our twenty-five years together, he has begun a project and has mastered each project. He has studied (and mastered) geology, astronomy, photography, rocketry, navigation, piloting, computer programming, aviation, dancing – yes, you can learn dance steps from a book! It's just the way he is. Bill's work as an Internal Medicine physician is stressful, so his projects have always been stress relievers.

Of course, I always wanted Bill to tackle theology. I went through many Bible Study classes and wanted him to join me. But he said theology would be the last and longest study of his life, and that once he started it, he'd never stop. Bill is a Christian baptized shortly after we married. He laughed saying he was a Christian with a "drug" problem. He had to be drug to church and drug to the Easter productions and drug to fellowship functions. He believed in God but did not have the relationship with our Heavenly Father that I knew he could have.

I myself was raised in the Simpsonville, Kentucky Baptist church, so for me, Christianity was just a way of life. Of course, during my college years and young adult life, I attended church sporadically, but there was never a tense moment that I wasn't in prayer. Once married and relocated to Mt. Sterling, Kentucky, we searched for a new church home. One Sunday morning, we visited Gateway Christian Church. Glenn Emery, a young, dynamic minister, spoke straight to my heart. Our daughters and I attended many Sundays and felt at home there. But Bill always had reasons for not attending; he was on call, or just got called out, or was up all night with a patient on Saturday. Except for our differing views toward religion, Bill and I were soul mates. We spent our every night and day together, and life was good.

In February, 2005, Bill and I sat in church together. Amid the dim lights and soft background hymns, we celebrated Communion, the part of worship I look forward to the most. We all bow our hearts to God in private prayer time. I don't know why, but I have always felt my prayers were heard more during that time than any other. That particular Sunday, I was praying for my family – I was especially praying for my daughter, Kimberly, who was going through a spiritual drought in her life, a difficult time when she questioned God. I prayed that God would squelch her doubt and show himself to her in a big way. I also prayed that Bill might have a daily relationship with our Lord Jesus Christ. "God, use me as a vessel to bring my family to you." Of course, I was thinking, "God, you tell me, and I'll tell them." But that was MY plan. God's plan is beyond our understanding. He sees the big picture and knows what works in our lives. I tell you of my prayer because it's where my story really begins.

Chapter 2

Dreams and Rainbows

"The thief comes only to steal and kill and destroy; I have come that they may have life, and have it to the full." John 10:10

Being a nurse married to a doctor certainly has its advantages, a quick diagnosis with quick treatment being one. Not that we ever needed it. Both Bill and I were exceptionally healthy for our ages of fifty-two and forty-nine, and we were both in great physical shape. We hiked regularly, went on scuba diving trips every year, were avid boaters and could even hang with our seventeen, twenty-one and twenty-three year old daughters on the ski slopes each year. We knew a healthy lifestyle would lead to a long and happy retirement. As an internist, Bill could clearly see a difference in the retirement lifestyles of those patients who stayed physically fit and those who did not. We knew we wanted an active retirement.

Early Tuesday morning, Mike Ginn saw me in his office before he started seeing his scheduled patients. I quickly jumped up on his examining table and smiled as I told him of my increasing pain and casually reminded him to look for growth in the small gallstones he'd seen in me a few years earlier. Minutes into the exam the small-talk stopped, and Mike excused himself from the room. He returned shortly with Bill to review the testing. The preliminary sonogram showed a pancreatic mass of 4.6cm. Bill called our daughters to let them know that we were going for further testing at the local hospital a mile down the road. A CT Scan confirmed the diagnosis. I had a pancreatic mass.

Our youngest daughter, Kimberly, had joined us in the hospital and stood in the Radiology lobby as Bill and I held each other and cried. She looked into our eyes, "Oh, Mom, Dad," rested her head on our shoulders and cried with us. My diagnosis came on her seventeenth birthday, the summer before her senior year in high school. My heart wept for her. Our lives changed.

With the diagnosis, we found ourselves as "patients" not medical practitioners. Terrified and bewildered, we stood in the lobby among some of Bill's patients who witnessed their confident, compassionate doctor transformed into a man convulsed by grief crying uncontrollably for his wife. Their awkward consolations, words of hope, offers of prayers for their physician, for me and our family humbled us.

I'm not a worrier, and I am definitely not a crier. Call me tough or cold, but crying is just too awkward for my German heritage. Standing in the lobby, I told myself and Bill and Kimberly, "I will *not* worry until I know a final diagnosis. I will not worry until it's necessary." But Bill had already seen our future flash before his eyes, "I wish I didn't know about these things, but I do." Little did I know that this would be the year that I would learn to cry.

Our other two daughters, Jenifer and Stephanie, met us at home. Jenifer, the oldest, was surprisingly calm. Leaning over mugs of hot tea, we all sat at the kitchen table and talked. I can't remember Jenifer ever telling me about her dreams, but she told me of an amazing dream she'd had the night before. "Mom, we were all sitting in a hospital room, and no one was talking. You were lying in a hospital bed, and we were sad and were just looking at you. No one said what was wrong, but we all knew you had cancer. I stood up from my chair and went over to your bed and sat down beside you and took your hand and said, 'God wants me to tell you that you're going to be okay.' "

Trembling, Jenifer continued, "Mom, I started to call you and tell you about my dream before I left for work this morning, but I didn't call because I didn't want to scare you. But today,

7

when Dad called me from Mike's office and said you were going for testing at the hospital, I knew you had cancer. Mom, you're going to get through this. You're going to be okay." We rested our empty mugs on the table, joined hands and prayed thanking God for his compassion and asking for His healing hand.

Finding a mass is just one part of the diagnostic process; biopsy follows to determine if the mass is benign or malignant. My biopsy was scheduled for Thursday morning in Lexington just thirty-five miles away where one of Bill's colleagues would do the testing. My life had always been so positive, so uneventful, so non-disastrous that it was hard to imagine the worst with this tumor. Though my prayers were constant, I was not an alarmist. I reassured Bill that I was not going to worry about this mass until I knew for certain what it was. I didn't want my sisters or daughters or anyone else to come for my biopsy. I didn't want to make a big deal of this thing in case it was nothing. I didn't even call Glenn Emery, my minister, but I did e-mail him, just to let him know what was happening and to ask him for prayer. That's all I felt compelled to do.

On Thursday morning as Bill and I sat in the pre-op area waiting to be called for the biopsy, I smiled contented it was just the two of us – no big fuss. Then it occurred to me -- Bill was going to have to go through this all alone. I'd be sedated, and he'd be sitting in the waiting room alone. What a mistake. I hadn't considered his needs – the needs of the man I love who suffered more than I did at that time. At that moment, I saw

Glenn walk in the room. He extended his hand to Bill and hugged me; he prayed with us and sat with Bill while other doctors tended to me. That Glenn had opened his email at 8:00 A.M. instead of his normal 4:00 P.M. "mail time" was a real God-thing. The Lord specifically placed Glenn in our lives to be with Bill that morning; the news was not good.

I had two diagnoses that day. A ruptured ovarian cyst which had bled into my abdomen caused the pain that had brought me in for the original sonogram. The second test confirmed adenocarcinoma, malignant cancer of the pancreas.

On the drive home, we sat in stunned silence. I had a virulent cancer and faced a painful death. Neither of us said a word for a long time until I said, "Now – it's time to cry." And both of us collapsed into primal sorrow. I prayed out loud, "God! Tell me what's going to happen! Live or die? I need to know, and I need to know now." I was emphatic, "If cancer's going to consume my life, I need to know now! My daughters! My daughters! Oh, God! I have to prepare my daughters. Tell me!" I needed to know God's will for my life because I wasn't going to my grave kicking and screaming. I wanted to leave lying in the arms of God, not fighting him. Comforting words from my grandmother's favorite poem calmed me; I could hear her reading the final stanza of "Thanatopsis" to me:

> So live, that when thy summons comes to join
> The innumerable caravan, which moves
> To that mysterious realm, where each shall take

His chamber in the silent halls of death,
Thou go not like the quarry-slave at the night
Scourged to his dungeon, but, sustained and soothed
By an unfaltering trust approach, thy grave
Like those who wrap the drapery of his couch
About him and lies down to pleasant dreams. (73-81)

Five minutes onto Interstate 64 and still in tears, I looked out my window to see a magnificent rainbow brilliant against the clear blue sky. It arched across the earth in front of us. As we slipped closer to home, we saw that it was a double rainbow. I stopped crying. Bill said, "Well, Honey, there's your answer." I felt the peace of God, and I knew I was going to be okay – whatever okay was.

That was the last time I cried about my cancer for a long, long time. Why wouldn't I be okay? God had sent me a dream and a rainbow. What else did I need to know that He had his arms around me?

I think God sends us signs to make us stronger for His glory, so that when the world sees a bold Christian face tragedy and suffering, He and His kingdom are glorified. In Anne Graham Lotz's *Just Give Me Jesus*, she says that if all is going right in our life, it is only natural that we can be "kind, thoughtful, happy and loving." However, if we are going through a crisis or trying time and "we are still kind, thoughtful, happy and loving," then the world sits up and takes notice. The behavior becomes supernatural and the glory of the Lord is "revealed in us" (183).

Chapter 3

The Journey Begins

"And we know that in all things God works for the good of those who love him, who have been called according to his purpose." Romans 8:28

We immediately scheduled an appointment with an oncologist who said that surgery is the best way to treat pancreatic cancer. "I'm referring you to a surgical team at the University of Cincinnati," Dr. Stephen Schindler said. "They specialize in pancreatic cancer treatment and surgery. My nurse has scheduled your surgery for June 16th, one week from today." I was excited about the surgery; the thought of chemotherapy didn't even bother me. I cheerfully awaited the opportunity to be cancer free.

Since Cincinnati, Ohio is a large city with a variety of things to do, and it's a ninety-minute drive from our house, Bill and I decided to make the most of our trip to the hospital. We would do some shopping, check into our motel, go for our pre-op doctor's visit and then maybe catch a movie that evening. On the way, we stopped at The Florence Mall for some last-minute shopping. I needed some house shoes for walking around the hospital, and I needed some mascara. Then I'd be done shopping. I picked out a pair of slippers and headed for the cosmetic department.

At the counter, a cordial dark-haired lady smiled, "May I help you?"

"Yes, thank you. I need one tube of waterproof brown-black mascara, please."

She reached under the counter, got the mascara and handed it to me. "Where are you going that you don't want anyone to see you cry?"

Her boldness shocked me. "Actually, I'm going to the hospital." Why had she asked such a question? It was June. I buy waterproof mascara every June for swimming. No one had ever asked me such a question when I bought mascara before.

"Are you going to the hospital for you?" she asked.

"Yes, actually I'm having surgery," I said quietly.

"What for?" she continued.

Her persistence surprised me, but I whispered slowly, "I have pancreatic cancer."

Suddenly, the fear was real. I'd never spoken the words. This pleasant woman, this total stranger was the first person who heard me say "Cancer. Pancreatic cancer."

She reached over the counter, hugged me and told me she would pray for my successful surgery. I humbly thanked her and left the counter knowing I'd just been touched by an angel. I kept thinking of the ladder for angels "…and behold a ladder set up on the earth and the top of it reached to heaven: and behold the angels of God ascending and descending on it "(*New International Version* Gen. 28.12).

Since the University Hospital provides hotel accommodations for patients' families, we booked a four-night stay so Bill and my daughters could switch off while caring for me post surgery. We checked in and then went next door for our pre-op consult with the team of surgeons. We came prepared with our list of ten questions. How long would I be in the hospital? How long would I be in the ICU? What was the exact procedure? We figured our planning would facilitate a quick pre-op meeting so that we'd have time for a movie before calling it a night.

The head surgeon, Dr. Mathews, entered the conference room, sat down and quickly asked if we had any questions. Silence. I looked to Bill who was in charge of the consult. He couldn't speak. He fought back tears. I laid my hand on his knee, reached for his list of questions, and started asking them one by one. Embarrassed to break down in front of a team of professional colleagues, Bill merely nodded his head as we listened to the answers.   I hated what I had done to him, my hero, my lead man. In our many years together, nothing had ever rattled him like this. My cancer had devastated his world, a world he no longer controlled. My disease was destroying his core being.

The meeting lasted almost an hour. These brilliant men quoted horrible statistics, probabilities and outcomes. They would first perform a laparoscopy to search for metastasis. If they found metastasis, they would abort the surgery intended to remove my diseased pancreas.

Although Bill and I already knew the statistics of pancreatic cancer, our knowledge had never been personalized. The onslaught was too real, too powerful. We had entered the consultation as a doctor's wife and a fellow colleague. We crawled out as a cancer patient and a terrified husband.

Shaken, we wandered through long corridors, "No, it's this way to the hotel, isn't it?" "I don't know, I don't know the way." A hospital volunteer who had passed us earlier kindly led us to the exit.

In our hotel room, we held each other, deciphered what we'd been told, and we prayed. Privately, we each were planning for the worst while hoping for the best.

At six o'clock the next morning, we reentered the hospital. We spied my sisters and mother already sitting in the surgical unit waiting for us to arrive. My father had been sick and was unable to make the trip to Cincinnati, but the family kept him abreast of news through phone calls. I was surrounded by my family and close friends, all chatting and praying for me while awaiting our news. My dear friend, Anita, brought a journal for everyone to write in while I was in surgery. She knew I wouldn't want to miss anything:

> It's 7:00 a.m., and we're all waiting in the family waiting room. We've been praying for you all morning. -Jenifer

> 7:20 a.m. God is going to shape you and prepare you for His work. You will come out of this with greater strength and understanding…someday you will look back and see this as part of the path that made you who you became. Love , Terry

> 7:45 a.m. Our hearts and prayers are with you. The time is going so slow. The minutes seem like hours… Your strength makes us all strong. I love you, Pat

> 8:10 a.m. We're all here eating doughnuts. Wish you were with us. I can't wait to get this all behind us. Love you, Kim

> 8:20 a.m. We just got a call in the waiting room – they have started the laparoscopy! This was supposed to start at 7:30 so this had caused a few mixed emotions, a few tears and certainly many prayers. Anita

8:35 a.m. Greatest News ! The laparoscopy showed no metastasis. You are going into surgery right now. The entire waiting room burst into a cheer and everyone cried happy tears... I love you, Stephanie

8:35 a.m. We have found out that you go to surgery now. Bill took the phone call. He sat down next to me where we had been talking, put his hands over his face and cried – happy tears – no metastasis. Love, Terry

9:35 a.m.   The operating room called to say the surgery was going okay. Wish you were here eating Krispy Kreme Donuts with us! Anita

10:10 a.m. The doctors called Bill into the consultation room.   Glenn went with him. We are all anxiously awaiting the good news we have hoped for. Anita

10:30 a.m. Jenifer walked into the consult room to be with Bill. Anita

1:10 p.m. Toni, we are waiting for you to wake up in the recovery room. The news the doctors told us is not what we wanted to hear. Each person here has handled the news in their own special way. Sadness is thick as fog as we process what we have been dealt. Our love for you is evident in each tear and is manifest in each sob and hug. Your precious daughters have reacted just as their mother would have wanted. They have held each other up and together comforted their father. You should be so proud.   I can't wait to see what wonderful things God is going to do with your life, now. I am so proud to be with you on this journey. Love, Anita

During the surgery, the doctors discovered an inoperable mass wrapped around the main blood vessels that sustain life to the intestines. They aborted the surgery. It was a heart-breaking time for my family.

Amazingly, God was again at work in my life. I awoke from the anesthesia in the post-op recovery room. I could see the clock on the wall -- 12:00 p.m. Nurses scampered in and out of the room not noticing that I was awake. Over and over I struggled, "How did the surgery go?" but they ignored me. At 12:20, my voice a bit stronger, I asked again, "Were they able to do the surgery?" Again, no response from the medical staff. As one of the nurses passed my gurney, I reached out and grabbed her hand, "Was the surgery successful?"

"Just rest, Honey, and your doctor will be here to talk to you soon," and she quickly left the room.

Holding back tears, I thought the worst. "They didn't do the surgery. You hear it all the time, 'They opened her up, and she had so much metastasis that they just closed her back.'" The worst possible outcome. I didn't understand. I could feel an abdominal bandage. Had I even had surgery? I wanted to see my family – they would talk to me.

Orderlies finally wheeled me to my room. Bill was the first one through the door. "Tell me, Bill, what happened?"

He smoothed my hair from my forehead and gently told me that the surgeons were unable to remove the tumor.

"Then they actually did the surgery? I don't have metastasis?" I gleamed. "Oh, Bill, we can handle this." There was no metastasis. Still just one tumor. Praise God, "For in all things God is working for the good of those who love him and are called according to his purpose" (Rom. 8.28). God had used the post-op nurse to remind me of just how bad it could have been. I was happy just knowing that the cancer had not metastasized. I knew something good would come out of this – I just didn't know what.

In his book, *Where's God When it Hurts*, Phillip Yancey says if you're looking for God on this earth, you'll find him in the people of His church (181). I found that to be true. To wake in the hospital on day two and read the journal written by loving friends and family was so encouraging. I was just beginning to realize how important it would be to surround myself with Godly, hopeful and loving people as I faced this trial.

In times of crisis, it's hard to keep faith. I go through dark nights when I don't see God, and I can't feel Him. This happens to me mostly in times of physical pain. I feel such distance. I have to remember that pain and darkness are straight from Satan and he wants to steal my thoughts.

The more I allow emotion and feelings to take over my thoughts, the more my hope diminishes. Satan is the deceiver and will use whatever means possible to steal my faith. At my lowest times, I need my prayer/pocket cards. I have to distinguish between what is real and what is not.

Emotions are fleeting and changeable. The word of God is unchangeable, and I need to keep His word in my back pocket at all times.

These verses speak to me of faith because I have to hold onto His word even when I don't see the outcome or the answer at the time. I have to stand on the promises and not the premises, holding fast to His every word. I suggest that everyone make their own pocket cards to have in their time of need.

I knew I would need strength and encouragement to heal after surgery, so before we went to the hospital, I copied some of my favorite Bible verses to read while in the hospital. These pages were verses of hope, encouragement and peace which I read many times each day. They became invaluable to me. God knew I would need them.

Chapter 4

Adjusting My Sights

"Do not conform any longer to the pattern of this world, but be transformed by the renewing of your mind. Then you will be able to test and approve what God's will is—his good, pleasing and perfect will." Romans 12:2

Nothing can turn your world upside down like cancer. I quickly realized that the things I spent most of my time doing were the very things that mattered least to me. How did I let that happen? How had I let my life get so lopsided? I knew better. I had gone through this whole priority thing with Jenifer when she was a senior in high school. One afternoon I asked her to come into the kitchen and told her to bring a tablet and pencil with her. She looked at me strangely but found a writing tablet and pencil and stood in the doorway. I nodded, "Why don't you sit at the table?" Still unsure of my motives, she nevertheless listened carefully as I talked her through a self-discovery exercise.

"O.K., Honey, I'd like you to list all the activities, all the things that are important to you in the order of their importance."

"Mom? Why am I doing this? Why do I have to do it at all?"

"Because I said so," was not an appropriate answer, so I replied, "Well, I think God presents us with so many challenges and opportunities, I'd just like to know – no, I think I'd like you to know so that you can share with me what's really important to you. That's all."

After Jen finished her list, I asked her to rank by percentage where she was spending her time. "Mom? Look at this! I don't even know what to say!" She and I both learned that she spent the least amount of time doing what was most important to her and spent the most time doing the things least important. That evaluation helped her make changes. If I could help my daughter prioritize her life, why hadn't I done the same for myself before I was diagnosed with cancer?

For twenty years I worked as a nurse in my husband's internal medicine practice, but in 2000 I wanted to explore an Internet business with a business partner. Even though I enjoyed being current with technology and felt like a valuable working citizen, the part-time job cost thirty hours of my life each week. Cancer prioritized my life for me. On day one of my diagnosis, I sold the Internet business, dissolved the LLC and recaptured the thirty–plus hours I'd given to the company. My life changed, and I began ridding my life of aggravation.

As a nurse, I know how important positive attitude is in overcoming disease. Emotionally and psychologically, I craved the "positive" -- positive people, positive situations, positive conversations. Sadly, some long-time friends were shattered by my disease and drifted away distancing themselves from me with awkward phone calls. My Christian friends, however, rallied to my needs. During my long, difficult convalescence at home, they prepared homemade soups, complete evening dinners and delivered those precious meals each day. The mail also brought daily showers of hugs; each beautiful card encouraged me and reminded me of God's healing power. These positive, hopeful people nudged me ever so gently but steadily toward healing.

One afternoon, Bill brought home small index cards that were a gift from a distant friend whom I respected and admired, Keen Johnson. As so often happens in people's busy lives these days, our paths rarely crossed anymore. Surprised and delighted, I opened the package and read his short note:

Toni and Bill,

I'm sending you these duplicate packets of prayer cards – keep one packet on your nightstand, one in the car, and one in the bathroom (yes! why not?!!). Read them together three times a day every day. I know you'll feel closer to one another, closer to God and closer to healing.

With prayers and all good wishes for your recovery,

Keen

Bill and I began our daily readings that evening. We kept the cards in the car, on our nightstand and yes, in the bathroom. We were bathed in the word of God.

One evening, my dear friend, Elizabeth, came to visit. As she settled into the sofa next to me, she asked, "Toni, Dear, what type of music do you listen to? What artists do you enjoy most?"

I confessed, "Jimmy Buffet, mostly, but I also listen to John Prine and lots of 60s &70s…."

She laughed with me, then said, "Let me just leave some inspirational music with you." She handed me a gift bag of Christian music CDs. I'd always liked praise and worship music, but once I started listening to the healing music CDs, I was delightfully surprised at how much I enjoyed it. In the mornings, I listened to *Selah* while I stretched and exercised. Meditation and exercise helped me stay both physically and emotionally healthy.

Elizabeth taught me to meditate with the healing music and to listen to God. So often my prayers were, "Give me, give me, thank you, thank you, I need," and so on. I had never listened for God's answer. I had never learned to be still and hear the word of God. The music trained my ear, filled my heart and opened my soul to God's message. I praised God for placing people in my life who were showing me how to heal.

To bolster a consistent positive attitude so essential to my fight, I focused on my spiritual life, on other people, or just looking to the future – not on myself. Daily, as I consciously considered what was good and what was right, the Apostle Paul often stood next to me, his words reinforcing my determination to guard my heart:

> Do not worry about anything but be thankful and pray to God about everything, and the peace of God which surpasses all our understanding will guard your hearts and minds. Finally, keep your thoughts on things that are noble, things that are just, things that are pure and lovely and are of good report, things that are of virtue and that are praiseworthy – meditate on these things. Doing so will bring you the peace that comes only from God (Phil. 4.6-9).

In my "pre-cancer" life, I could easily lose myself in negative thoughts. Someone would upset me, a movie would scare me, the evening news would be gruesome, my daughters would have drama in their lives, and my evening and sleeping hours would be fretful. Unaware, in my "pre-cancer life," I dwelled in negativity. In my "post-cancer" life, however, I changed the negativity into positive action and peaceful acceptance. I didn't want to be left out of my daughters' lives nor shelter myself from anything abrasive; I stayed mindful of God and His word, and I learned to be at peace with my situation. It was God's peace. I was learning to lay my problems at the feet of God.

I recall when I stopped focusing on my pain and suffering, knowing that I could drown in either. As soon as Linda Burton, a good friend and survivor of liver cancer, shared her "five minute rule" with me, I decided that this rule was a good one to follow. On a really bad day, I allotted myself five minutes to dwell on myself - to think about my situation, to think about my losses, to bemoan my shortcomings, to experience pain, to succumb to suffering. I cried for five minutes. Any more time was a pity-party, and such self-indulgence would render me emotionally, physically and spiritually bereft.

Years ago while learning to snow ski, my instructor told me that when skiing down a hill, I needed to keep my sights on the downhill path. If I saw a mogul or hole, I should just glance at it and know it's there, but not look at it too long. If I did, I would fall right in it! He told me to keep my focus on my downhill path. That was good, solid advice on and off the slopes.

Being newly diagnosed with inoperable cancer, I needed a positive attitude, a strong spirit and unfaltering determination to maintain both; I also needed hope. Not the hope of this world, but the hope of God. Hope that I could feel in my soul. The hope of knowing that what can happen, will happen. I reminded myself that a cancer diagnosis is not a death sentence. "Every form of cancer presently known to men has been survived "(Barry 24). I would not let the survival rates for pancreatic cancer frighten me. After all, those statistics were compiled on people much older and much sicker than I. I accepted the challenge of getting myself into the one percent survival group!

The immune system is one structure the body has to inherently fight off disease. God gave me a strong immune system that had always kept my body healthy. In my "post-cancer" life, I had to strengthen that system physically and emotionally. To increase my physical strength, I changed my diet, I purged the cupboards of sweets, chips and junk food and ate only healthy meats, fruits and vegetables. I also exercised as much as possible; long walks with Bill healed me both physically and emotionally.

So that I could direct all my energies to strengthening my immune system, I also knew that I had to salve an emotional wound I'd carried around for twenty years -- a wound from another time in my life from an argument with a very close family member which caused years of stressfulness. My hurt pride prevented me from forgiving her – I falsely believed that forgiving her "let her win," "let her off the hook." Yes, forgiveness is difficult, but non-forgiveness is a sin and a burden to the soul – neither of which I could bear any longer. So I forgave her. That's what I did. I got over it. The wound healed; the stress disappeared. I had prayed for many years that God would soften my heart toward her and help me learn forgiveness, but the battle continued. It wasn't until I learned to pray for her that my heart was softened, and the wound was healed. God's a big God -- He restored *agape* love and resurrected forgiveness in me.

Chapter 5

Brokenhearted Hope

"Do not be anxious about anything, but in everything, by prayer and petition, with thanksgiving, present your requests to God. And the peace of God, which transcends all understanding, will guard your hearts and your minds in Christ Jesus. Finally, brothers, whatever is true, whatever is noble, whatever is right, whatever is pure, whatever is lovely, whatever is admirable—if anything is excellent or praiseworthy—think about such things." Philippians 4:6-8

Dr. John Cronin is such a jovial guy. It was hard to believe he'd been an oncologist for 30 years. You'd think dealing with such a heartbreaking profession everyday would harden one's outer core but not his. He had been a highly respected friend of Bill's for many years, and now he was my doctor.

At Dr. Cronin's office, we revamped my surgical plan. Since there was still no treatment to kill an existing tumor other than surgically removing it, we decided to pursue chemotherapy and radiation in an effort to prevent new tumor growth or metastasis. We hoped this treatment would shrink the tumor enough to attempt another surgery.

Chemo and radiation treatments would be physically stressful and technically difficult since the Lexington Clinic Cancer Center was forty-five minutes from my home. Even though I did not work, I knew that recovering from surgery and being sick from treatments would try my physical and emotional soul. Violent vomiting from the chemo would wrack my incision - a large cut straight down from my sternum which branched left and right toward each hip bone.

Thank God for my family and friends because it took all of them to care for me during those many long months of chemotherapy and radiation treatments. Back at home, my mother came to stay with me the first week after surgery and that helped a lot. Bill was working full time and acting as nurse at night. He was worn out. The chemo treatments started in late June. Rosemary Barnes, a long-time friend, worked at the Lexington Clinic and drove me to my 8:00 AM chemotherapy treatments every Monday. We had great talks on the way to treatments. She's such a consoling, compassionate person that I shared with her both the good and bad of my life. Every Monday morning, we laughed or cried all the way to Lexington.

Caring for their mom after surgery and during cancer treatments was difficult for my daughters. Kim, my youngest, had just started her senior year of high school. Although she took me to treatments and stayed home with me in late June and early July, her summer was tightly scheduled, and school started in early August. A varsity soccer player, she had two soccer practices most days, in early morning and late evening. Kim was also involved in the Junior Miss program which required daily practices in July to prepare for an August 10th performance. She threatened to withdraw from Junior Miss more than once, but I insisted that she participate. Jenifer, my oldest daughter was a newlywed with a new highly demanding career in pharmaceutical sales. Jenifer and Ryan, her husband, lived five minutes away and were a great support in the evenings, but they couldn't help during the day. So, I was left in the lap of my middle child, Stephanie, who eagerly and lovingly accepted the challenge. A sophomore at the University of Kentucky, she cut back her college hours to the minimum of twelve hours and took most of those hours as online courses. She substituted at Bill's office, working on accounts receivable and payroll; she worked at home, paying all our personal bills and relieving me of many household duties. Stephanie drove me home from my Monday morning chemotherapy treatments and then went to Bill's office to work the rest of the day. She took care of me on the days I was sick: Monday morning I received chemo; Tuesday evening I was nauseated; Wednesday, Thursday and Friday I vomited; Saturday I was better; Sunday was a great day, just in time for Monday morning treatment.

It was a long, hot, challenging summer since the summer heat and chemo don't mix. The heat exacerbated the vomiting, but Bill kept me out of the hospital by starting IVs and running fluids on me at home. I was a past ICU nurse and Bill was a physician, so we both knew how to work intravenous fluids. We both admit, however, that it took him a while to regain his skills.

Bill's first attempt at starting an IV after so many years was not uneventful. He came home with all the necessary equipment and declared, "Kim, I hereby declare you my assistant." There was some joking about the difference between "assistant" and "assassin." But Kim assured both of us, "Dad, Mom, I can handle it. I've seen lots of horror movies."

Bill prepped my skin and then pulled the needle out of the sheath. He looked at Kim and then he looked at me, and I knew instantly this was going to hurt. Memories of the pain we nursing students inflicted upon our mothers in college during our "How to Start an IV" class flashed across my mind. I took a visible sigh of relief as Bill easily inserted the needle into my vein with the very first stick. That was the last thing that went right.

Bill knew how to start an IV, he was just unfamiliar with the new IV bags and tube apparatus. Kim, of course, had never seen the equipment. Kim held the tubing but didn't know to shut the fluids off using the stopcock. Bill didn't know how to regulate the connecting tubing. He fussed and carried on for about fifteen minutes before giving up. Blood and IV fluids spurted all over my hair, the bed, the carpet and Bill. They wrangled themselves and me out of the bedroom, put me in the car and took me to the emergency room where I received fluids for dehydration while Bill humbly received IV training from the ER nurse.

That summer was different from other summers also because I wasn't working outside the home. For the first time in my life, I actually had time to myself. I delved into reading. So many friends had sent or brought me great reading materials – daily devotionals, books on healing, an assortment of encouraging religious resources. I loved it! I could actually set aside time for reading the word of God. I learned so much and realized that even though I'd been a Christian all my life, I knew very little about religion. I'd relied on others to teach me rather than discovering God's word on my own. I had begun a new journey into the life of Christ and I loved it! In my daily Bible study, I rediscovered James 5:14-15:

> Is anyone among you sick? Let him call for the elders of the church and let them pray over him, anointing him with oil in the name of the Lord. And

the prayer of faith will save the sick and the Lord will raise him up. And if he has committed sins, he will be forgiven.

One Sunday after services, I did just that. My church elders, family and friends escorted me into the adjacent small chapel. They invited me to sit in a chair and then formed two concentric prayer circles around me. The elders offered prayers, followed by prayers from my loved ones. The Bible doesn't say do this and you have an 80% better chance; it says DO this and you'll be healed. My faith and their prayerful petitions filled me with confidence and a trust beyond my understanding. I knew I'd be "okay."

The months of chemotherapy and radiation treatments were grueling, but they worked. Throughout the treatments, I felt like a little duck on the water, bobbing my head "yes" to everything the doctors told me to do, but beneath the surface I paddled and prayed constantly. In October 2005, four months after my first surgery, I was scheduled for my second surgery – this time with a world renowned physician, Dr. John Cameron of Johns Hopkins Hospital. Ranked as one of the best pancreatic surgeons in the world, if anyone could remove my tumor, I knew Dr. Cameron would. He and his team of surgeons were doing some miraculous things with the Whipple operation. I desperately wanted this tumor out of my body, and I was finally connected with the man who could do it.

To get to Johns Hopkins, however, we had to fly to Baltimore, take a 30-minute taxi ride to the hotel near the harbor area, then another 15-minute taxi ride to the hospital. Bill and his buddy Mike Ginn (who had originally diagnosed me through ultrasound) took off work for the week. Mike's wife, Jenny, my oldest two daughters, Jenifer and Stephanie, and of course our minister, Glenn Emery went with us. Melanie, my craziest sidekick, also flew up for the day of surgery. Bill was adamant that my mother and sisters stay behind. Besides the expense of travel for them, Bill knew he couldn't be responsible for their safety and travel around the town while trying to care for me. Of course, he was right.

With everything a "go," my spirits were high before this second surgery. I'd been through the normal pre-operative procedures and was lying in the pre-op holding bay. I'd given loved ones and friends my last kisses and hugs and was alone when Dr. Cameron came in for last-minute instructions.

"Don't worry, Mrs. Roberts, we'll take good care of you. If anything goes wrong, we'll stop the surgery and not take extraordinary risks."

"No," I said, "do not stop the surgery. I need you to get this tumor out!"

"Well," he explained, "if you start to hemorrhage or have other complications we'll stop the surgery."

I sat straight up in the bed and grabbed his hand. "No, Dr. Cameron, do not stop until you have this tumor out."

He slowly pulled his hand from mine, stared at me, then disappeared behind the curtain. He knew what I meant. I would rather die on the operating table than have a painful death from inoperable cancer. I felt like he was my last hope.

As I lay on the table waiting to be wheeled into surgery, I thought about the previous four months. Maybe we can't really appreciate the good in our lives until some bad creeps in. I had spent more time on my knees praying, had felt God's presence and sometimes his distance, had cried more deeply, had laughed with greater joy, had loved every person and had appreciated every experience life had given me. I'd grown more in the last four months than I had in the previous forty-nine years.

The surgery went poorly. Tissues were so boggy from past surgery and radiation, I hemorrhaged on the operating table. Again they couldn't remove the tumor. Again they closed me up. Again I was inoperable. This had been my last chance to remove the tumor.

The day after that surgery was the worst day of my life. During their morning rounds, doctors told me that I could have no further surgery; that I had already taken the maximum dose of radiation; that the chemo would not kill this tumor – it would only prevent new cell growth. One of the interns spoke up, "Possibly in a year or so the tissues might heal enough to try the surgery again. . . ." But the flash of hope he inspired faded quickly as I saw senior physicians look at him disapprovingly.

"Mrs. Roberts," the lead surgeon said, "although we have no surgical alternatives for you, clinical trials might be a possibility." They knew I wouldn't be here in a year. It was a general consensus that they didn't know what we were going to do.

That day I lay silently in self-prescribed isolation -- motionless, without hope, without prayer. I did not want to talk to anyone; I did not want to see anyone. Worst of all, I couldn't muster a single word in prayer for myself. Friends and family called; I did not answer the phone. Prior to this surgery, I had placed all my hope in the famous surgeon, the famous hospital, the new technique. I'd spent weeks letting my hope slip from God to man, and when man failed (because man does fail), I lost all hope. As evening lurched into darkness, I plunged into an abyss of utter hopelessness. Every waking moment was a struggle.

My Bible studies had told me that when you are unable to pray for yourself, the Holy Spirit will intercede for you and lift you up in prayer. As the night wore on, I began to feel that intercession. I felt many prayers going up for me. A blanket of peace comforted my soul. By the next morning, I was better. I was praying again, but I prayed a prayer of total surrender. I ceased bargaining with God and surrendered my life to Him. "If you have work for me to do on this earth, then you'll find a way to get this tumor out. And if not, then you must have something bigger and better in store for me than I can even imagine – Heaven! Well," I said to myself, "that will just be okay, too." I felt at peace – the peace that results from God's presence – the peace that calms, reassures and comforts. When everything around me was dark and void, the Lord restored me with hope for the future and the perseverance to take it one day at a time. Again, I knew I would be okay whatever "okay" was.

My private room at Johns Hopkins was complete with comfortable cherry furnishings and, more importantly, high-speed Internet connection. Bill and my nephew Camm, who was now my primary doctor and Bill's medical practice partner, stayed online constantly looking for new treatments for my cancer. Bill finally connected with a pancreatic surgeon at Sinai Hospital of Baltimore which happened to be nearby. They decided that I'd be a candidate for a new treatment called CyberKnife. Because the treatment was still in trials and not offered by Johns Hopkins Hospital, Bill was getting anxious and on the third hospital day, he threw me a towel and told me, "Get up, get a shower, get walking; we're getting out of here." I was ready to leave, too. It seemed that every morning I heard condolences rather than a plan. Sure enough, on day four, Bill pushed my wheelchair through the airport while I clutched an abdominal pillow and prayed for a soft landing and an easy two-hour car ride home from the airport. My fresh incision felt every bump, every lurch of the car. But Bill was right; we needed to get home so we could start laying out our next plan of treatment. Time was a-wasting.

Chapter 6

A Questioning Belief

"… acknowledge the God of your father, and serve him with wholehearted devotion and with a willing mind, for the LORD searches every heart and understands every motive behind the thoughts. If you seek him, he will be found by you; but if you forsake him, he will reject you forever." 1 Chronicles 28:9

In a small town, news travels fast. When I returned from Johns Hopkins, everyone in Mt. Sterling, Kentucky already knew the news. More than one hundred cards and letters confirmed that hundreds of people in five different states prayed for me while I was in the hospital. This outpouring of care was all good for me, but it made Bill's life difficult.

After twenty-five years of practicing medicine in Mt. Sterling, Bill had one of the largest clinics in town. Since my daughter, Stephanie, stayed with me at home, Bill went back to work as soon as we returned from Baltimore. Time at the office was devastatingly difficult for him – not his treatment of his patients, but his having to answer their hourly, daily queries about me, "How's Toni?" Although he certainly appreciated everyone's concern and their offerings of prayers, the additional stress eventually turned to anger. He didn't want to think about me and my cancer while he was at work. Work provided no escape from the facts -- the finality of our life together. One evening as we snuggled on the sofa, Bill admitted that each time he entered an exam room, he struggled to fight back tears. He finally dealt with his patients' well-wishes by putting up a sign, "Please don't ask about Toni because I can't take care of YOU if I have to think about her!" The sign helped very little; Bill's concerned patients still asked about his wife whom they'd also known for the past twenty-five years.

Bill became very protective of me. He screened phone calls, and if I looked tired, he said, "Toni's sleeping now." When visitors came, he would suggest, "Please keep your visit short; Toni tires very easily." He spent his every waking minute with me; he tended my physical wounds, bathed me, helped me change into my clothes, read with me, "delivered" my mail, held me close during quiet and difficult hours. Bill's difficulties, however, were more complicated than my own.

From the hour that I was first diagnosed with pancreatic cancer, Bill silently fought his own emotional, spiritual and physical battles. After twenty-five years of marriage, he was looking forward to retirement, grandchildren and the future we'd always planned together. We weren't rich, but we'd set aside money by doing without the things we could have had, knowing that those sacrifices would allow us an earlier retirement together. That future was being destroyed, and Bill felt robbed. Of course, he knew how this disease progressed into a 1% survival rate or a quick, grueling death. He shouldered everything by himself, and the titanic responsibilities wore him down. He provided physical care, emotional support as my devoted, loving husband. He prayed, pleaded with God, yet his prayers remained unanswered. All of his efforts – his knowledge, skills, devotion, passion wrought no change in my disease – his gallant efforts only compromised his spiritual and physical being. In Michael S. Barry's book, *A Reason for Hope,* Dr. Harold Koenig says, "Having cancer can be a difficult experience even for persons with deep religious faith. For those struggling with their faith, however, the burden of this disease can be enormous "(qtd.in Barry 13). Bill was struggling. Ironically, I walked around smiling as if everything were okay. His friends asked, "Is Toni in denial? Does she not know the statistics? Have you not told her?"

Bill envied my calmness, and he also envied the calm faith of Mary, one of his patients in end-stage breast cancer, in hospice with two months to live. One slow afternoon in Bill's office, Bill met with Mary, his last appointment of the day. As she stepped down from the examination table, she asked Bill if he were a man of faith. "Do you believe in God?"

"Yes."

"You think God can heal me, don't you?"

"Yes, I believe God can do anything He wants to do."

"Well, do you think the sun will come up tomorrow?"

"No, I *know* the sun will come up tomorrow."

"You see, Doctor Bill, that's the difference," she explained. "That's the faith I have in *knowing* that God will heal me." Bill sat silent as Mary continued. "My faith assures me that what I hope for will happen." Mary gathered her jacket, purse and car keys, and as she opened the door to leave, she smiled, "You know, we're building a new home right now – I fully expect to live in it."

Bill admired her faith. He wanted that faith but didn't know how to get it. Bill prayed from the very beginning of my cancer, but he could not comprehend why his prayers remained unanswered. "Should I pray differently? Should I plead for something besides Toni's healing? How should I pray? What words? What more can I pray for? Does God hear me?"

Bill's emotional and spiritual trials were also complicated by his own physical symptoms. Bill had a real connection

41

with me that was not only soulful, but physical. When I was pregnant, he also gained weight. And now that I was sick, he was physically ill, also. He experienced excruciating abdominal cramping, bowel changes, and other physical symptoms which could have been very serious. An endoscopy showed gastritis and Irritable Bowel Syndrome both caused by worry and stress. By Bill's standards, not to worry was not to care. He didn't know how to lay his worries at the feet of God. He wanted to be a godly man with the faith that could move mountains. Daily, he read the Bible and Christian books trying to find peace, but anger instead of grace consumed him.

Bill quietly carried his stress for long weeks, but then he would explode in unpredictable, unintentional, uncontrollable anger. He exposed his fears, his pain, with bitter remarks about God's cruelty. "Where's God's mercy?" he challenged. "How can a *loving* God let people suffer?" On a quiet, pleasant afternoon drive through the country, as we listened to music and viewed the beautiful fall colors, Bill unexpectedly turned off the music, stopped the car, looked at me and asked, "How can a God of love do something like this to us? Toni, don't you understand what's going on? Do you not know your prognosis? God let his followers who gave up everything for him back in the Bible days die horrible deaths and be crucified. He didn't help them. What makes you think He's going to save you?" Tearfully, he said, "If God wants me to believe in Him, He's going to have to first show me a miracle of healing."

It was hard for me to watch Bill struggle with such painful emotions—this exceptional, loving man directed all his anger toward God. For the believer, a miracle is not necessary, and for the non-believer, a miracle is never enough. My husband was watching his dreams and everything he'd worked for slowly fade. I knew Bill believed in God, but his embittered outbursts were nothing he could control. He hated everything.

Bill loved challenging my friends and spiritual confidantes, Anita, Vickie and Linda, who wore their armor well when Bill grilled them. I could tell when Bill was frustrated with his reading because he'd suggest we call Anita and take her out to dinner just so he could drill her on Biblical issues that didn't "suit" him. Linda often brought food over, or she stopped by for a quick, "Hi, Toni. Just wanted to give you a quick hug before I head to the store. Can I get you anything?" Bill seized these moments. "Well, what about this-or-that Bible verse? O.K., so why do you think God let all those missionaries die?"

Linda finally told him one day, "Bill, you need to get that chip off your shoulder before you can ever understand the love of God." She was right. Bill's scientific mind did not condone the notion that some things just didn't have a concrete answer. How would my illness glorify God? The standard Christian answer," You just have to have faith" frustrated him even more than not understanding.

Bill has several close buddies who are strong Christians, but they didn't have the answers Bill was seeking. They are comfortable not knowing all the answers and being content to wait until heaven to discover the answers to difficult questions. Vickie's husband, Charlie, is one of Bill's best friends, but Charlie didn't enjoy Bill's Biblical interrogation as much as Vickie did. We went on trips with them and spent good amounts of time discussing the Scriptures. A Sunday school teacher for many years, Vickie set aside time each day for Bible study. She devoted patient hours discussing obscure areas of theology with Bill. Collectively, she, Anita and Linda helped Bill transform his head knowledge into heart knowledge. Because Bill sought God with all his heart and because God tells us, "You will seek me and find me when you seek me with all your heart "(Jer. 29. 13), I didn't worry about Bill's spirituality.

In October 2005, only a handful of hospitals in the United States provided CyberKnife for pancreatic cancer. The day we arrived home from Johns Hopkins, Bill began making phone calls. A hospital in California, my first choice, turned me down saying I was too high risk, and therefore, a poor candidate for the procedure. Sinai Hospital, however, agreed to treat me. However, we collided head-on with our health insurance carrier who initially denied pre-approval for the CyberKnife procedure still in clinical trials. After weeks of negotiating, haggling, and begging, the company signed off on the experimental treatment.

Doctors explained that with the "radiosurgery," I'd possibly see an immediate thirty percent reduction in tumor size and that the radiation would continue to work over the next nine to twelve months, reducing the tumor a little at a time. The doctors also told me the tumor would always be there, until surgically removed, but that it would eventually "scar in" and die. Excited and hopeful, I was thankful that God had led us to it.

On Tuesday, Wednesday and Friday of Thanksgiving week, 2005, I received CyberKnife treatments. In other times, we celebrated Thanksgiving with thirty or so family members all sitting down together at my house to a huge potluck dinner followed by an afternoon of laughter and sharing. But Bill and I had traveled to Baltimore by ourselves, and we observed Thanksgiving alone in our hotel room since the hotel restaurant and all the nearby restaurants were closed. Despite our Spartan holiday, we were thankful to have each other. When we felt life had disappointed us, it was because we had focused on what we'd lost, what we didn't have. Despair cannot exist when we focus on our blessings instead of our losses.

We were so thankful to have Dr. Cammual Suttor as Bill's new partner. Camm was my nephew, and he'd just graduated from Dartmouth as an internist and had started working as Bill's partner about a year earlier. Bill could take the time off to be with me without having to worry about who was going to take care of his patients. Camm stepped up whenever needed; he relieved Bill of additional stress that he simply couldn't bear.

Christmas time soon arrived and with it came the job of decorating for the season. We normally put up a large outdoor display -- Santa and sleigh, lighted angels and thousands of tree lights. This year, I changed our entire approach to decorating. We had a three-by-ten foot vinyl sign made which Bill and the girls erected on the hilly roadside near our house. The huge black sign with white letters read, "BELIEVE." We were amazed and humbled by people's responses to our simple decoration. All winter long, people called about the sign. One man called to say he was coming home from work, struggling with a difficulty in his life, and as he rounded the hill beside my house, he saw my sign which gave him the answer he needed. Others told me that the sign prompted quick, sweet prayers for me and prayers for themselves asking for God's wisdom and grace.

Oddly, the sign made me question what I believed as well. When I pulled out of my drive each day, rounded the hill and saw the sign, I asked myself, "Well, Toni, just what do you believe?" I had to do more than just believe in God. I had to know that He was my Jehovah Rapha, the one who heals. I had to know that He wanted to heal me: "Praise the Lord, O my soul, and forget not all his benefits - who forgives all your sins and heals all your diseases" (Ps. 103. 2-3).

With these short excursions past my sign, I came to believe that God is in control. HE controls EVERYTHING that comes into our lives - every situation, every relationship, every circumstance is either allowed or decreed by God, and He'll use it for our good. He will take the situation, and in the quickest manner possible, use it to do the most good for the most people to bring them to his glory (Ingram 128). This doesn't mean that every situation will have a happy ending. That's not God's goal for our lives -- to make us happy. His goal is to make us more Christ-like. To make us His own.

Christmas came and went with bushels of emotion – we were joyful for the season but saddened with the thought that it might be my last. I always loved Christmas and loved overdoing the gift thing for my daughters; it's just what we did, be it right or wrong. This Christmas, even though I tried to limit my gifting, my husband had gone all out. Bill and I normally exchange a gift or two, but as we passed out the gifts Christmas morning, I realized that Bill had purchased every gift he'd ever wanted me to have. It was exciting at first to get such extravagant gifts. Ryan, our new son-in-law, new to our Christmas celebration, exclaimed, "Wow! You're making out like a bandit! You must have been a good girl this year!" As I slowly realized that I was the only person in the room opening presents, the girls tried to joke about the obvious. They glanced at each other with embarrassed sadness knowing that their father was acknowledging this Christmas as my last Christmas with them.

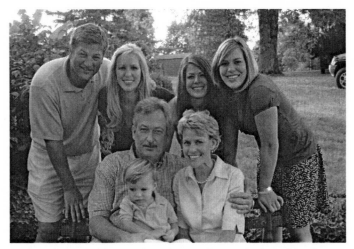

Toni with her family. (Back) Ryan, Jenifer, Kimberly and Stephanie. (Front) Bill and Toni holding their grandson, Will. September, 2008. Photograph by Terry Ethington

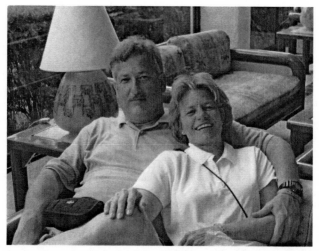

Bill and Toni on a scuba diving trip in Cozumel, Mexico. April, 2005.

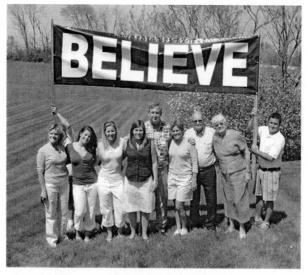

Family gathering around the "Believe" sign to celebrate a cancer-free
Toni! April, 2006.

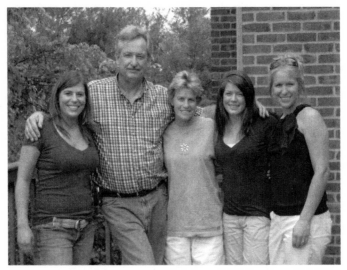

Toni with her family on Father's Day, 2008. (L-R) Stephanie, Bill, Toni, Kimberly and Jenifer.

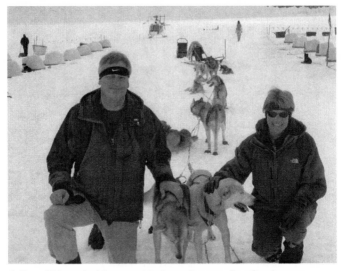

Bill and Toni sledding in Alaska only months after her recovery. June, 2006

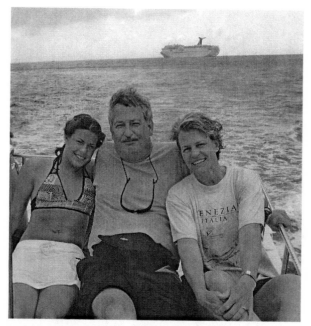

Kimberly, Bill and Toni on a dive trip in Cozumel, Mexico.
April, 2005

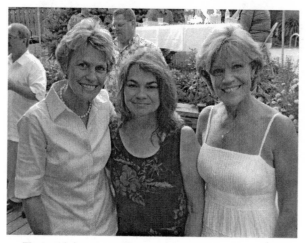

Toni with her sisters Terry and Pat. September, 2008.

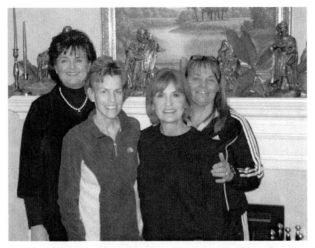

Anita, Toni, Vicki and Linda after a Bible Study. December, 2008

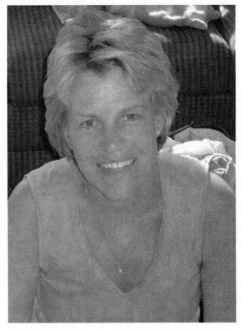

Toni boating at Cave Run Lake the week before she was re-diagnosed with cancer. May, 2008.

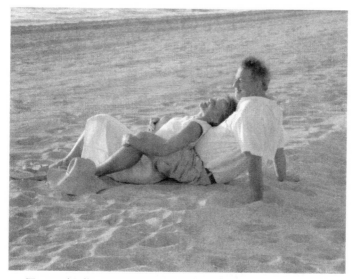

Toni and Bill on Captiva Island in Florida just before her 2006
remission. April, 2006. Photograph by Terry Ethington

Chapter 7

Life's Reconciliation

"He gives strength to the weary and increases the power of the weak. But those who hope in the LORD will renew their strength. They will soar on wings like eagles; they will run and not grow weary, they will walk and not be faint."   Isaiah 40: 29-31

It was a long winter. I resumed chemotherapy in early December, the week after I came home from my Cyber Knife procedure, and by late January 2006, the chemicals were wearing on me. My declining lab values were indicative of how I looked and how I felt. My bone marrow was taking a beating and couldn't keep up with the chemo damage. In late January, a

CT scan showed no change in my tumor. The Cyber Knife had proven ineffective – the tumor had not shrunk. Instead, I had developed an enlarged spleen from the tumor blocking a duct and was hospitalized to receive a platelet transfusion. Clearly, not the best results, but through everything we'd been through, Bill and I learned to be thankful, and we were thankful that the tumor hadn't grown or metastasized to other organs.

I discovered during that time what "living it from the inside out" really meant. I walked in my bathroom one morning and saw an unfamiliar gray face in the mirror. As I touched my reflection, I winced, barely able to look at her -- this thin, frail woman with pallid skin and patchy hair trumpeted a "call to arms." "Toni, it's time you started living your life from the inside out!" Turning this way and that, I came to believe that the new appearance was more attractive than the old, and I smiled. God was carrying me through life every day. He put a smile of faith on my face, a smile that radiated from my soul outward.

Bill was also having a change of heart. He was getting ready for work one morning and praying for me while standing in the shower. Still steamy from his shower and wrapped in a towel, he came into our bedroom where I was resting and said, "It was like a wave came over me - so hard it almost knocked me down! Toni, I feel like God just spoke to me! 'Don't call out to me!' He said, 'you don't even know who I am!'"

No, God doesn't hear the prayers of people who doubt Him. That morning, Bill realized how weak his faith was. He admired people who had strong faith, people who believed God and the promises given in His word. Bill wanted that faith. As the water cascaded down his body, he realized that doubt resonated in all his prayers. Scripture tells us that faith is essential to the unlimited power of prayer. "But when he asks, he must believe and not doubt, because he who doubts is like a wave of the sea, and tossed by the wind"(Jas. 1.6). Beth Moore states in her workbook, *Believing God,* that we need to believe God is who He says he is, and we need to believe God can do what he says He can do (9). Bill realized he believed in God, but he did not believe God.

Bill started rereading his Bible. He read everything anew. He bought an extra book for every book of the Bible to help him understand what he was reading. He also bought an extra Bible and highlighted in blue and flagged everything in it that he didn't understand and that he didn't agree with. Before long, his entire Bible was highlighted in blue and flagged with markers. Bill was more miserable than when he started. He didn't understand. Why did the Bible say that slaves should be good to their masters? Why didn't God just say, "Don't have slaves…we're all equal?" Why did it mandate women shouldn't talk in church?

Every Sunday, Bill walked into Bible study class skeptical and full of questions. He was prepared and willing to debate every topic. He wanted answers! Betty Joe, our minister's wife, answered him, "Read on." So he did. He read deeply groping for answers to unanswered questions. How can someone's death glorify God? Why did Jesus have to die? Ever so slowly, Bill realized that every time he faulted the Bible, the fault was within his own heart. His heart needed to change – not the words of the Bible.

Bill spent four to six hours a day all through the winter of 2005 and early spring 2006 reading Christian books, watching sermons online, staying in the Word, and building his faith. He was so thirsty for the Word of God. Bill wanted to make sense of my illness; he wanted to know why bad things happen to good people. Why did cancer happen to me, his cherished wife? I used to joke with him that it wasn't **that** bad (it would have been worse had one of our children had cancer), and I wasn't **that** good. As the Word of God permeated his heart, Bill began to understand God's promise for our lives. "For my thoughts are not your thoughts, neither are your ways my ways, declares the LORD. As the heavens are higher than the earth, so are my ways higher than your ways and my thoughts than your thoughts" (Isa. 55.8-9).

Everyone who knows Bill noticed how much he had changed. He developed a deepened love for people. His patients spoke to me of his new tenderness and compassion. His friends noticed a new generosity, and his family sensed a more humble and kindhearted person. He now dragged **me** to church. He wanted to go on Sundays, even when I didn't feel like going. My cancer drained him emotionally, physically and spiritually, and now he was finding inner peace – just at a time when things became physically more difficult for me.

By early March 2006 I was a metabolic mess. In a composite blood test of thirty-five lab values, thirty of the values were seriously abnormal. I stayed home most of the time. On rare outings, however, I wore a face mask due to my low white blood count. I felt wasted and looked worse than ever. But through that time, I actually felt nearest to my God. I called on the Lord sincerely, and knew that He would be close to me (Ps. 145.18).

At this time, my dear friend Anita encouraged me to go on an Emmaus Walk, a three-day spiritual retreat for women sponsored by the Methodist churches. I wanted to go but didn't think I'd be well enough to leave home for that long. With no other treatment option to prevent metastases except chemotherapy, I was reluctant to miss a single dose. Two weeks before the retreat, however, my oncologist told me he had cancelled further chemotherapy -- it had become too toxic for my body. I was at a point where nothing was working, and there was nothing left to try.

Tormented thoughts muddled my mind. Stopping chemotherapy allowed me to feel well enough to attend the Emmaus Walk, but terminating chemo meant there was nothing else we could do to rid my body of cancer. All that was left was to pray for God's healing. Funny, how you run the gamut and end up doing what you did in the beginning – just praying. I had lived in a state of constant prayer for many months. Why didn't God answer me? What was His plan for my life?

I know you've heard that unanswered prayer is sometimes an answer in itself. Well it is. I discovered that God intentionally delays answer to prayer so that we have time to try to fix our problems all by ourselves. Bill and I had called on everyone we knew. We'd tried everything we knew to do and had exhausted all our own resources. In the end, we realized that all we had was God (Lotz, *Just Give* 203-204). And that's when we realized that "the grace of God was all we needed because His strength would be made perfect in our weakness" (2 Cor. 12. 9).

Once I reconciled myself to the end of chemotherapy and what that indicated, I was eager to go on the Emmaus Walk. As it turned out, the retreat was a time of great spiritual renewal. I felt fine the whole time. I made many dear friends that weekend with whom I laughed and cried and bonded. We shared our hearts and minds, but I didn't tell them that I had cancer. The retreat wasn't about me or my illness or my anguish. It was about my relationship with God. At the Emmaus Walk, I fully surrendered my life to God's will. I knew I was going to be okay – whatever "okay" was. God was in control.

After the Walk's concluding evening service, I needed to talk to someone about my cancer. I had planned to mention it to one of the clergy so he would pray for healing with me.

That night I approached Merelene, a lay person who sat at the table with me all weekend. I don't know why I chose her – I think it was another God-thing. She told me that she, too, was a cancer survivor. She'd had lung cancer just a year earlier. She reminded me that the darkness in our lives comes from Satan. Satan comes to destroy us, but Jesus comes to heal and give life to the full (John 10: 10). Merelene told me to go home and find a room where I could have privacy. Then she offered golden advice: "Toni, you go into your private room, and you yell at Satan; you command him to get out of your body; and you demand that he leave you alone. And you do this in the name of Jesus Christ."

The day after I came home from the Emmaus Walk, I did just what she said. I was already used to going into my closet, closing the door and getting on my knees in prayer to God. But in my closet this day, and in the darkness, I stood in the name of God. With tears streaming down my face, I railed, "Satan! Do you hear me? I command you to leave me alone! 'Get thee behind me.' You get away from me and take your damnation and your darkness with you. I am a child of God – you will not devour me – you will not control my life! I have given my life to my Lord and Savior – you will never take it!" Then, I turned on the closet lights and packed my clothes for Florida.

We left on our family vacation that very day. I felt so much better. When I left for the Emmaus Walk, I took fifteen pills every day; when I returned home, I was taking ten pills a day.

I needed fewer and fewer pills for pain, nausea and digestion. My energy improved, and my color returned to normal. I'd endured chemotherapy for nine months, and being free of it left me feeling energetic and in good health.

Chapter 8

Waste Not a Single Sorrow

"Cast all your anxiety on him because he cares for you. Be self-controlled and alert. Your enemy the devil prowls around like a roaring lion looking for someone to devour. Resist him, standing firm in the faith, because you know that your brothers throughout the world are undergoing the same kind of sufferings. And the God of all grace, who called you to his eternal glory in Christ, after you have suffered a little while, will himself restore you and make you strong, firm and steadfast." 1Peter 5:7-10

Easter arrived late in spring of 2006, two weeks after we returned from Florida. I'd been busy the months of March and April preparing to be in our church's seventeenth annual Easter production, *The Living Last Supper.* I don't sing well, but I volunteered to be an "extra" in this beautiful musical drama which drew large crowds every year. Still, I had to learn the music and words even if I only mouthed the parts when I couldn't reach the high notes. It was such a privilege to be part of such a devoted, spiritual group.

My next set of follow-up tests was scheduled for Monday, the week before Easter. A full month had passed since I'd seen my oncologist, so if the cancer were going to grow, it would certainly be visible now! I went in for the tests Monday and expected my results sometime on Wednesday.

I was to have a PET Scan and a CT Scan. The previous tests in January had showed no change. Doctors who performed the November CyberKnife treatment told me the tumor would always be visible on my CT Scan, but at some point, if the treatment worked for me, the tumor would die and become an area of scarred dead tumor cells. We would be able to tell if the tumor were viable (alive) by looking at the new PET scan because it would show areas of tumor activity. Often, the PET scan gave false positives due to inflammation in the area. To be quite honest, I was neither excited nor worried about these tests because the readings all seemed so "iffy." I wasn't sure anyone would be able to put all this together for a complete test result.

I believed additional testing would be required anyway, so I wasn't going to let test results ruin my day.

And it was a big day. Wednesday evening was our first of five performances of the Easter drama. Bill usually takes Wednesday afternoons off, so we went hiking in the Daniel Boone National Forest with some friends. After a three-hour hike, we raced home to shower for the Wednesday evening performance. I drove to church in my own car because the cast gathered two hours before each performance to prepare our hearts and minds for the presentation. It was a time of laughter, prayer and fellowship which drew us closer with each performance. I was glad that the test results had not come that day. If there were bad news, I certainly did not want to change the atmosphere nor the mood of the performers.

While I was at the church, Bill went to his office to see if he had received my test results. He ran into the church an hour before the performance was to begin. He was crying and waving papers in the air when he found me in the fellowship hall. "Toni! Look! Look! They're all normal! Every test – every one is normal!" It was as if I had never had cancer. There was no false positive. There was no sign of a tumor – dead or alive – on the CT Scan. There was no dead tumor presenting as scar tissue. There was no sign of previous surgical intervention. The scans were *so* normal that Bill called the radiologist to see if we actually had the right test results. The radiologist had also questioned the test results and had already had the tests read again for confirmation. It was real. My cancer was gone. God didn't want there to be any question or "iffy" results. I felt like I had just had my third surgery, and this time it was by the great Physician himself. Through God's abiding grace, my pancreatic tumor was gone.

How was I healed? Was it the medicine? The CyberKnife? A miracle? I don't know, but it doesn't matter. What I do know is that God had been at work in my life. God is in control of all things, and He makes things happen for His glory. He has a way of taking ordinary people and transforming them into great vessels of faith, vessels fit for His use, ones that can testify and display His glory to the watching world (Lotz, *Why?* 9). Michael Barry tells us that miracles do happen. They don't happen every time and they don't happen to everyone, but they happen for a reason (58). Miracles let us see God at work on this Earth. God wants us to see answers to our prayers because they glorify Him and build our faith.

What timing! Easter – when our eyes are already opened to the miracle of the resurrection. We had prayed for eleven months, and now, the evening of our Easter production, my tests showed I was healed – cancer free. Hundreds of people who had been praying for me would gather in the church that evening to witness an answer to prayer. God may not come early, but He never comes too late.

God's timing was perfect for many reasons. Physically, if my surgeries had been successful, like I had prayed, the surgical team would have removed my pancreas, and I would have had many residual problems. I would probably have been on an insulin pump and required heavy medication for the rest of my life. As it is, now, I have no residual problems. Spiritually, if my surgery had been successful, we would have been thankful and we would have felt blessed, but we would not have had time to grow in the Lord. And spiritual growth takes time. God was the potter who molded us, changed our lives and shaped us in Christ.

When I prayed for my family's spiritual growth back in the winter of 2005, I never dreamed what was ahead for us. How was it that I prayed over and over for our Christian growth, and then as soon as God started us on that path, I was on my knees begging Him to take it from me? God took me through trials and through periods of brokenness. My family was broken, and I was broken, too. At times along the path, I cried out, "Abba, Father. Take this. I want your will in my life. I want your will to be my will because I know I can't do it without you." God worked in my life in deeper and more wonderful ways than I had ever imagined. God healed me physically, and he healed Bill spiritually. That's how my God worked in my life.

Wow! What now? What do I do with this? My cancer was gone.

Joyce Myers, the author and Christian motivational speaker, tells us that God gives us experiences that show His love, and He gives us talents to share those experiences. When we don't share what God has given us, we defy the purpose of what we're called to do. We waste God's gift to us. I did not want to waste a joy – I did not want to waste a single sorrow if any could bear testimony to God's abiding love and grace. God comforts us so that we can comfort others. He uses us as a living testimony to others. How could I share what had happened in my life? God opened the door for my work.

Within two weeks of my healing, the Lord's Ladies at Gateway Christian Church asked me to speak at their annual women's banquet. I immediately thought of twenty reasons why I couldn't. "I've never done public speaking. I'd be horrible. I don't know what to say – I once had cancer, now I don't." I didn't feel bold enough to claim myself as a miracle of God, yet I knew a miracle sent me into remission. How would I share my testimony with others?

Doris, a friend from church, reminded me of a promise I'd made months earlier. I promised her that if I were ever healed, I'd yell it from the mountain tops. She made it very clear that I had no reason not to testify to the glory of God. That evening while I told Bill why I shouldn't give the talk, he recited my favorite Scripture, Romans 8:28– the very verse which had given me so much hope since day one. "And we know that in all things God works for the good of those who love him, who have been called according to His purpose. " I had never heard the last part, "…who have been called according to His purpose." How had I missed that? For the first time in my life, I heard God calling me to do His work. Acts 3:13 says, "When they saw the courage of Peter and John and realized that they were unschooled, ordinary men, they were astonished and they took note that these men had been with Jesus" (Acts 3.13). That's how God works. He takes ordinary people and gives them a testimony and the courage to share it with others. There was no longer a question as to whether I would speak in front of a group. God had healed me for a reason, and I wasn't going to waste his work. I began my speaking ministry.

God allowed me to touch thousands of lives. People from the Relay for Life, the Women's Health Forum and other women's civic organizations invited me to speak. So many churches asked me to speak, and most of those churches asked that Bill and I both give our testimonies. They wanted to hear about Bill's spiritual healing as well as my physical healing. Word travels fast, and I think someone must have posted my name somewhere because I received five or six phone calls every month from people who had pancreatic cancer. Some were very sick and in late stages; others were newly diagnosed. I talked to each of them for hours. Sometimes, I became their email pen pal. We discussed feelings as much as the medical treatments, and I gained great satisfaction being able to talk openly about our cancers. People with cancer need to talk. They need to share both the good and the bad.

I'm so thankful for the opportunities God gave us to share our testimony. I never understood how people could stand up and say how thankful they were that they'd had cancer. Maybe I'm just not there, yet. I just know that God empowered me – He empowered Bill – to speak. We grew as Christians and for the first time, our thoughts and hearts were in sync with each other and with God.

Chapter 9

Embracing the Shadow

"For my thoughts are not your thoughts, neither are your ways my ways," declares the LORD. "As the heavens are higher than the earth, so are my ways higher than your ways and my thoughts than your thoughts." Isaiah 55:8-9

Bill and I started traveling and doing all the things we'd always wanted to do. I felt wonderful and needed no medication. We went to Alaska, traveled to Florida, hiked Glacier Park and the Smokey Mountains, and reveled in our health and opportunities to enjoy life.

When I had cancer, I longed to see the birth of my grandchild. Joyfully, on March 9th, 2007, with the extended family on both sides present, Jenifer gave birth to our first grandchild, Will. Two months later when Jenifer returned to work, I kept Will two days every week—such a gift to hold my wiggly, perfect, cooing grandson. I cherish those times.

Life was so good for Bill and me. We regularly attended church; Bill participated heartily and happily in Sunday and Wednesday evening Bible study groups. We were both studying God's word and were loving life. It was the happiest time of my life. God-loving people surrounded me, and God's will guided me. I was working for His glory and loving the opportunity to do so -- and so many opportunities came our way. The *700 Club*, a national television audience, invited us to give our testimony on the show in November 2007. How exciting to be aired with a Christian television program, knowing that thousands of people could receive hope in their own trials through watching us and others that shared God's promise on that TV show. God kept opening doors and connecting us with people whom we helped and who helped us. I'm convinced that nothing happens by coincidence. Every person, circumstance and situation occurs in life as a result of God's sovereign plan for our lives.

We went to our doctor regularly for follow-up appointments and continued to test for reoccurrence of cancer. By May 2008, my oncologist believed I was fine and set up my next follow-up appointment for six months. Bill encouraged him to do one more CT scan because I was having some vague back pain. Bill was right. My cancer had returned.

On May 30th, 2008 doctors found a new tumor in my pancreas, close to where the original one had occurred. Almost three years to the day after my first diagnosis, I again had cancer. This time we were on top of it -- we knew just what to do. Bill immediately contacted the pancreatic surgeon and head of CyberKnife at Sinai Hospital in Baltimore. My CT was sent to them for a re-read, and they agreed I was a candidate for CyberKnife again. I was to have the procedure in two weeks. I was okay with the new diagnosis. I focused on how much I'd grown from my first round with cancer and almost looked forward to the opportunity of growing as a Christian and knowing that God was close to those who suffered. I loved being obedient to God and couldn't wait to see how he was going to work in my life this time.

I went to Sinai in early June 2008 for the CyberKnife treatment. Since I'd had little difficulty with the first treatment in November 2005, I wasn't that nervous about it. The first CyberKnife was three treatments over a four day period. In Summer 2008, I had five treatments, five days straight, Monday through Friday. It was agony. I was so sick, unable to eat anything without severe nausea and stomach cramping with each meager meal. But we made it through. I say "we" because Bill, as usual, was steadfast every step of the way.

The high dose of radiation from CyberKnife was too much. I did not recover from the treatment and a few days after we returned home, I was hospitalized. During that seven days, while doctors tried to restore my bowel function and treat the dehydration, they discovered that my cancer had grown. A new CT scan showed a second tumor in my peritoneum, an area just outside the pancreas, and many other sites which my doctor suspected were probably cancer cells also. "Well, Toni, Bill, knowing how this disease progresses, I think six months is a reasonable prognosis." This prognosis hit me harder than the same words I'd heard after the first aborted surgery in 2005. Side effects from the CyberKnife treatments and the physical agony of the previous days exaggerated my anguish. Pain exaggerates everything.

These CT findings were one more God-thing in my life. Three doctors had not seen the additional tumors. My first CT in May 2008 showed one tumor. The same CT images sent to Sinai to be over-read as a pre-testing procedure for my CyberKnife treatment verified only one tumor. A second on-site CT Scan at Sinai prior to CyberKnife treatment found one tumor. Two tests and three radiologists confirmed that I had one tumor. The significance of this missed diagnosis is that patients with multiple tumors are not eligible for CyberKnife. That I had a second CyberKnife was astonishing—another God-thing. He wanted me to have the second CyberKnife treatment.

Things change, life changes, but God's love is constant. I handle this cancer differently than I did in 2005. Why? Bill is such a different person. He is not as physically or mentally stressed. On the dark days when I am mentally or physically down, Bill reminds me of God's love for us and of all the good and positive things in our lives. He knows God is working in our lives today just as He was in 2005. Bill is now the godly leader of our family that I always wanted and always needed.

My very personal relationship with God keeps me positive. How could I get through such a trial without Him? I'm so thankful that He took the time to prune my life and challenge me to become a better Christian. Cancer, yes, cancer made Bill and me seek God and crave His closeness in ways that we could not have known without my cancer.

Cancer: Round #2 is just beginning. The blows are tougher this time. I have more pain. Pain makes it hard to stay positive. My body and my mind are Satan's battleground where he pummels me daily. I'm a little angry, but I keep Romans 12:2 in my pocket: "Do not conform any longer to the pattern of this world, but be transformed by the renewing of your mind. Then you will be able to test and approve what God's will is—His good, pleasing and perfect will." I pray daily that the Holy Spirit quiet my mind and keep me from despair. I handle disappointment biblically and quickly to thwart Satan, the deceiver, the enemy. I do not dwell on what I'm missing or losing – Satan wants me to drown myself in desolation. I cannot and will not let Satan win this championship round.

In May 2008, I was initially embarrassed by the reoccurrence of my cancer. I'd spent two years giving my testimony at churches and organizations with Bill giving his testimony of faith and of my healing, testimonies of how God had miraculously put all things in place for my healing. Almost three years to the day, I have cancer again. How could I ever speak to those groups again? Why did God miraculously heal me and then allow it to return?

Had I not prayed enough? Had I been backsliding? Is that what I'd done? Had I taken my new life for granted and not continued to honor God and give Him the glory? Perhaps. Scripture tells us, "Later Jesus found him at the temple and said to him, 'See you are well again. Stop sinning or something worse may happen to you'" (John 5.14). The man went away and told the Jews that it was Jesus who had made him well.

Time with my Christian friends showed me that Satan launches fierce insurgencies on people who do God's work. Satan attacks Christians whose minds he intends to destroy, whose hearts he intends to shred, whose trust in God he intends to dispel. A good friend, Jim Curley, told me, "Toni, look what God has allowed you and Bill to do! All your letters to people you don't know but who needed your help. All your testimonials to inspire others! Your healing in 2005 was a miracle and still is a miracle. Why is it less of a miracle because your cancer returned now?"

"Okay," I said. "Absolutely! Satan is not going to tarnish my miracle nor any others God might work. The Lord works miracles all the time; what He does once, He can do again."

Am I mad? Yes. That this cancer came back doesn't seem fair. I'm a better Christian now. I see God's love and His work all around me. I have a grandchild that I want to have time to know and time for him to know me. But, I'm mad. And that's okay. Even Job in the Bible praised God when his children were killed, when his wife died, when all his worldly possessions were taken from him. He had disease and pain, yet he still loved God. At one point Job expressed his own anger, "Lord, why have you set me as Your target?" (Job 7.20). God responded, "Wait a minute, Job. Where were you when I laid the foundations of the earth?" (Job 38.4). That's how I feel right now.

Like Job, I feel angry, but God answers me, "Hey, Toni, where were you when I healed your disease? Did you not see Me at that time? Why would I want anything less for you now?" I know God is working for my good (Rom 8.28), but I erred in thinking that God is working for my happiness. When God's plan differs from my own, I get mad.

So . . . what am I going to do with this anger? Who am I mad at? If I were mad at God, I'd have to assume He caused my cancer when He didn't. Anger is okay when it's used as God intended. God gave us the emotion of anger for a reason.

Jesus was angry at the money changers and the merchants in the temple because they had turned his Father's house into a den of craft and mercantilism (Matt. 21.12). Satan tells me to keep my emotions bottled up. When Satan belittles my miracle, I scream, "Satan go away from me!" But mostly, I try to use my anger constructively. I write about it and talk about it. I focus on the abundant love in my life – the love I've given and the love I've received. It's hard to love and to be angry at the same time.

As we mature as Christians, we slowly learn how to turn things over to God. Sometimes we think we surrender everything, but we really don't. I surrendered my first cancer in 2005, but fear stood in my way this time. Releasing control, even when we're surrendering it to God Almighty, is tentative, difficult. But through submission to God's will comes perfect peace. Not through Bill's work nor my own will my illness be solved. Bill can only take care of symptoms; he cannot change the course of my disease nor can I. We have such peace in knowing we don't *have* to solve it. I can't. Bill can't. Together, we handed it over to God, the divine Pilot whose flight plan is wiser and grander and more beautiful than my own. There is no better knowledge than that sweet harmonious, celestial peace that comes of God's will. I pray that God will guide the medical team in finding treatment for my disease.

During my cancer, I came to know Herb Atkins, a retired missionary who lived in Florida and who sent weekly inspirational e-mails to many of his friends. My friend, Anita Gray, forwarded just one of his weekly emails to me, and I was hooked. Anita had told Herb about my cancer when I was just recovering from my first failed surgery. I knew from the beginning that Herb was a wise and Godly man. From my first reply to one of Herb's emails, we became great friends, spiritual allies. Bill had just begun his Bible studies, and Herb suggested texts for Bill to read and ways that I could help Bill search for his faith. Herb sent me inspiring verses just when I needed them most; he kept me focused on the good and on what God COULD do instead of what I couldn't do. Herb was jubilant when I was healed of cancer that April in 2006. Ironically, in June Herb e-mailed me to tell me that he had pancreatic cancer. He was seventy-two years old and was otherwise in good health, but his cancer had metastasized, and he grew very sick very quickly. His email asked his friends to pray for his comfort and peace, not healing. He reminded us, "I have fought the good fight, I have finished the race, I have kept the faith" (2 Tim. 4.7). In July 2006, Herb died.

I've wondered if a different prayer would have changed Herb's life. How do we know God's will? When is it time to fight and pray for healing? When is it time to pray for peace in our lives, that peace that only comes from God? I think Herb focused on eternity not on this world; I think Herb knew God's plan for his life.

God has three answers to prayer. First, He'll answer, "Yes!" That's when we see that miracles happen all the time – the ones God wants us to see because they answer our prayers, build our faith and glorify Him. Sometimes He answers, "No, not yet," and that's when we see God's perfect timing. During my first cancer in 2005, God rendered me utterly dependent upon Him. And I'm there again, surrendering my illness to Him, laying it at His feet knowing that I cannot cure myself. And sometimes God answers, "No, I have a better plan for your life." That answer reminds us that God is faithful; He is omniscient. We only see our narrow view of life. God sees into the future knowing the timeline of our lives and what's best for our future. He, alone, knows our future.

I go through rough times when I feel like I have lost everything good and precious. We go to our houseboat; I can only think about the fun we used to have. I miss the times when the girls were young, and we played in the water, pulled them on water skies, tubed with them behind the boat. Such wonderful days on the lake. I want those times with my grandchildren. We walk through the woods in Daniel Boone National Forest, and I think of the fun we had hiking with our daughters, and I remember their gleeful excitement of finding turtles. I remember their "Shhhh! Shhhhhh! Whisper!" when watching deer. I dwell on family photographs of our snow skiing trips, knowing I won't be able to snow ski this year. I know I'm slipping into a place that I don't want to go. After much prayer, God answers me.

I realize that images of the good times shouldn't make me sad. They should bring me great joy knowing that I was able to have those good times. I should be happy knowing that I provided those opportunities to my children, that I was able to bring joy into their lives. So, I don't despair in thoughts of loss, but I sit content and joyful and grateful for the opportunities I've had in my life.

Bill and I are okay. We've come through the anger and are now trying to settle on the other side. We love one another completely, we know one another intimately, we trust one another utterly; we love God faithfully, we know God profoundly, we trust God utterly. Knowing that God's plan is perfect, who's to say that what's in store for me is not better than what I had planned or imagined or prayed for?

I have walked through the valley and may soon stand in the shadow of death. There was a time I would have feared that darkness, but now I feel the growing need to embrace the shadow – to let the shadow comfort me as the darkness of evening brings a time of rest from the trials of a long, hard day. When the shadow comforts me, I will take my rest in the arms of Jesus. Until that time comes, I will continue to work on my spiritual and physical healing. I want to love more deeply than I've ever loved before. I will continue to write because it's a form of therapy for me. Whether I'm writing of anger or love, writing brings me peace with any issue. I'll continue to stay in close contact with my dear friends and loved ones who keep me lifted to God daily. I'm so fortunate to be loved by so many and to have such love for my family and friends. Lastly, I will continue to physically fight for my recovery. I'm working with my medical team to seek trial studies for a cure. I'm getting out of bed on days when I'd rather sleep, I'm eating when I don't want to eat, and I'm walking each day to regain physical strength. Everything else is in God's hands. Most importantly, I'm laying my disease at the foot of God, surrendering everything to Him.

Bill was asked to speak at a small church one Sunday while the minister was on vacation. He was to speak on suffering. Bill brought a small candle and some fall foliage and placed it on the front of the podium. As he lit the candle, he began, "I do not claim to be an authority on suffering, but only one who has experience with suffering. Let's suppose one-third of the lights in this church represent all your material worth and physical possessions. Let's kill those lights." The ushers turned down the lights. "Now, let's presume the next one-third of the lights represent all your friends and family you've ever known. Please kill those lights." The room grew dimmer as the next third of the lights went out. "Alright. Now, let's presume this final light represents you, afflicted and suffering, just as in the book of Job. Please kill those lights now." And then there was darkness in the church. One small candle glowed at the altar and illuminated the entire church. Everyone sat transfixed. After a few seconds, Bill said, "Please turn on all the lights."

He looked at fellow Christians in the sanctuary, "How many of you saw the candle's light when all the lights were bright?" Not a single hand went up. "How many of us here see God when all the lights are bright in our lives? James 1:2 tells us to count your suffering as joy. Is it better to have gained the whole world and lost your soul? Count it pure joy if you have been so broken that you have turned it all over to God and have been able to see the candle of light that represents Christ. Most all of us can testify that we've grown more in Christ from our suffering than we ever did through prosperity. That's certainly been true for Toni and me."

I'm not going to waste my time asking, "Why me?" but instead I ask, "How can I use this illness to glorify God?" Though I live under the shadow of death, I rest in the blessed assurance of the grace of Christ.

God's goal for our lives is to grow in Christ, to serve Him, to aid the suffering and less fortunate, to relinquish ourselves to God's will, to spread God's Word, to love others, to love God, and to accept suffering as God's reminder, "Hey, I'm still here. And wow! Have I got a plan for you!"

Acknowledgements

There is never enough room to acknowledge those people who have shown their love and endless support for me and my family over the past few years. So many have taken their time to prepare meals, shuttle me to treatments, visit, call and send mailings showing their concern and encouragement and bringing real joy into my life. Sometimes it was the person who was inspired to send that one card that was exactly what I needed that day. Nothing is by coincidence; they were God-inspired.

Above all, I want to thank my God and Savior for his work in my life and his enduring comfort and guidance. Through my faith in Him I have been able to surrender my worries and have the peace of knowing that I am in His loving hands.

I thank Bill, my husband and best friend, for his patience and understanding of my need to write this book. Words cannot express my gratitude towards him and that is why I dedicated this book to him.

Many thanks to my editor, Gay Morrill. She helped me put to words what my heart was feeling when I couldn't. Betty Jones, a long-time friend, also used her professional abilities and helped me edit and complete the technical intricacies of writing my first book.

Without the help of my sister, Terry Ethington, I would have never completed this book. Her endless encouragement pushed me to go further. Since her early help, Terry has continued to drive an hour and a half from her home to mine to help me every week or so. She's a spiritual woman with a gift of wording that helped me find the right words and was a reminder to me of many occurrences since she was there -- living through my story with me.

I've been blessed with three girls who are beautiful both inside and out. They are the ones who initially pressed me to write this book. I thank Jenifer Steger, my oldest, for her advice and comfort. Our daily talks and heartfelt conversations have helped me stay strong spiritually and emotionally. Jenifer was married two months before my first diagnosis, and it's safe to say that her life has never been one of normalcy since her wedding. Her husband, Ryan, is a strong and compassionate person who is so dear to my heart. Nearly a year after my 2006 remission they had their first child, Will. Working full time, dealing with me, caring for her child, Jenifer is always overwhelmed yet stressing that she's not doing enough. Stephanie Roberts, my middle child, is the most practical and she's my "doer." It was Stephanie who physically cared for me after my hospitalizations. She stepped up to take care of my bookwork at home and in the office. She sacrificed her time and energy more than anyone. Kimberly is my youngest daughter, and I think my illness hit her the hardest. At her tender age of seventeen, she was forced to grow up quickly, many times making her own dish for senior banquets and attending events without me at her side. All three of my girls have been there for me in every way, comforting both me and their dad.

Even though my family lives over an hour away, I am very close to them. My sister and forever friend, Pat Carriss, has kept me focused and excited about my life. She is the most kind-hearted and giving person I know. Her visits and understanding have made my life better. My parents, Nancy and Elmo Ethington, have inspired me in other ways. Mom was diagnosed with kidney cancer in 2007. Though currently in remission, she has had several complications and my father has been ill as well. They live one and a half hours from me so it's difficult for either of us to make the drive to see each other. It's neat knowing the unconditional love that's between us. My parents and I have an understanding that we love each other and would be there if we could, but health reasons all around are limiting us to phone calls. I'm just thankful that I can still pick up the phone and know they're there.

Once you've been married longer than you've NOT been married, your in-laws are as loved as any family member. Bill and Jean Roberts have loved me and prayed for me, and I appreciate their support. My sister-in-law, Kathy Castle, and her husband, Bill, have both prayed for me and been a source of inspiration throughout my battle with cancer.

God gave me wonderful, spirit-filled friends who continually feed me the word and help me through my physically difficult times and my emotional draughts. I can't thank Anita Gray enough for being a best friend in every way. She manages to send me uplifting cards and books just when I need them. Anita is a strong Christian woman who always says just the right thing. She understands and is such a giving person, working as the hands and feet of Christ on earth. Linda Burton has been a blessing by showing up at the right times, offering to stay with me in the hospital or whatever I need. Melanie Terrell has been the friend who kept a smile on my face and in my heart. She was one who just knew what I needed and made herself available in an instant. Rosemary Barnes is a long-time friend who drove me to chemotherapy treatments in a different town. A special thanks to Georgia Gay who has been part of our family for 25 years—there are not words that can express my gratitude for everything she has done for our family. Elizabeth Evans has prayed for me and with me many times throughout my journey. Many friends have gone above and beyond to show their concern for me by frequently sending cards and making phone calls checking on me and offering their time for visits: Loree Detwieller, Pam Ritchie, Pat Peck, Carolyn Bentley, Sandy Lansdale and Judy Howard, just to name a few. To all my dear friends, I thank you for making my life easier and more fulfilled.

I want to thank Jim Curley for his deep, late night conversations on religion and spirituality with both of us. He is the one man who Bill admires for his critical thinking and vast knowledge of the Bible. He was the one person who could always keep Bill's focus on God in the right direction. Jim is a colon cancer survivor and was inimitable in his empathy and understanding of my situation after my surgeries. He and his wife, Tammy, have been invaluable to me.

Bill and I both have been fortunate to have couples who helped us through our journey. Mike and Jenny Ginn shut down their private company for a week to travel with us to Baltimore for my surgery. Vickie and Charlie Rice have been a God-send to us in many ways. Charlie has been an ear to Bill, allowing him to vent his frustrations and really befriending Bill at his most drained times. Vickie has spent countless hours doing everything from helping me edit my book to cooking for us and even coming over just to sit and talk. Ron and Nora Oliver are boating friends from a different town but stay in touch weekly offering their love and concern. Camm and Deb Suttor have cared so much for us and have made it possible for Bill to have time off of work to care for me. Sandy and Terry Thompson have been life-long friends who have been there for us every step of the way. Curt and Ann Steger are spirit-filled people who have encouraged us with God's word just when we needed it. To our boating friends at Cave Run Lake who have given us laughter and great memories, I thank you: Proc and Bobbie Caudill, Brent and Melanie Terrell, Lisa and Rob Whitt, Barbara Lyons, and Vivian and Jerry Beatty.

I've talked about God-things throughout this book. Cheryl Walz is just one of those God-things. We were great buddies in college but over the years we didn't see much of each other basically due to distance and time restraints of kids. As I was writing this book and looking for an editor, Cheryl came to Kentucky for a visit and consequently hooked me up with Gay, my editor. Cheryl knows me better than most and will always hold a big spot in my heart.

I thank my church family and my minister, Glenn Emery, for keeping me mindful of my goal on this earth which is to glorify God through all things. They have cooked meals, sent cards, visited and prayed with me. Though you are too many to mention, I pray that you know how much of an inspiration you've been to me.

Works Cited

Barry, Michael. *A Reason for Hope: Gaining Strength in Your Fight Against Cancer*. Colorado Springs: Cook Communications, 2004.

Bryant, William Cullen. *Thanatopsis. Yale Book of American Verse*. Ed. Thomas R. Lounsbury. New Haven: Yale UP, 1912. Reprint. *Poetry Archive*. December 2008 (http://www.poetry-archive.com/b/thanatopsis.html).

The Holy Bible, New International Version. Grand Rapids: Zondervan, 2002.

Ingram, Chip. *God as He Longs for You to See Him*. Grand Rapids: Baker, 2004.

Lotz, Anne Graham. *Just Give Me Jesus*. Nashville: Nelson, 2000.

_____. *Why? Trusting God When You Don't Understand.* Nashville: Nelson, 2000.

Moore, Beth. *Believing God: Experiencing a Fresh Explosion of Faith.* Nashville: Lifeway, 2002.

Yancey, Philip. *Where is God When It Hurts?* Grand Rapids: Zondervan, 1990.

CPSIA information can be obtained at www.ICGtesting.com
Printed in the USA
LVOW08s1326250416

485210LV00001B/18/P